BODYBUILDING, POWERLIFTING, AND HIIT

WHILE IN PRISON

THE MAX-INTENSITY, MAX-RECOVERY WAY FOR MAX-GAINS

BOBBY FOREVER

BODYBUILDING, POWERLIFTING, AND HIIT WHILE IN PRISON:

HEALTH & FITNESS, SPORTS & RECREATION

REVISION 0

COVER DESIGN BY: GERMANCREATIVE

 DISCLAIMER: THIS BOOK IS FOR ENTERTAINMENT PURPOSES AND I AM NOT YOUR TRAINER, HOWEVER PRIVILEGING THAT WOULD BE. I AM NOT LIABLE FOR ANY INJURIES OR HARM YOU SUSTAIN YOURSELF, WITH OR WITHOUT MEDICAL APPROVAL.

EDITION (03, 2021)

ISBN:9798712927449

NONFICTION > HEALTH & FITNESS > EXERCISE

NONFICTION > SPORTS & RECREATION > BODYBUILDING & WEIGHT TRAINING

CONTENTS

INTRODUCTION

If you're reading this book based on the title, then this book is dedicated to you, since I wish I could have had a simple, dive head-first book as this one. This book will attempt to help you check all the boxes of weightlifting and fitness. Of course, without all the fat. Enjoy!

HOW TO USE THIS BOOK

You will first calculate your calories and repetitions. Next, we'll look at the routines. Lastly, you will execute what's in this book. Or, for the more analytical person, read the nuts and bolts, plus the various myths of weightlifting.

PART ONE

DIVE HEAD-IN

CALORIE COUNTING & MACRONUTRIENTS

Calorie counting can be as easy as completing the Harris Benedict equation, which you'll find in page seven. Then, add or subtract calories depending on whether you want to gain or lose weight. 3,500 calories equal a pound, divided by 7 for the seven days in a week equal 500 calories a day, to increase or decrease your weight by a pound a week. So, if you want to go up or down a pound a week add or subtract 500 calories to your total daily calorie expenditure. Now, once you reach your desired weight, simply eat the calories for that weight.

MACRONUTRIENTS

Water, fat, carbohydrates, and protein are your macronutrients. Micronutrients are your vitamins, minerals, etc. Water equals 0 calories per gram, fat equals 9 calories per gram, carbohydrates equal 4 calories per gram, and protein equals 4 calories per gram. It doesn't matter what they are, they will always come out to those values.

Food is made from these macros and the difference between foods is in the content of these macros. Your recommended macros are 0.6 g of protein per pound of body weight. Note, you might have heard it's per lean pound, but the truth is it's much easier to work with poundage of goal weight since your body composition will gradually change as a result of this program to more muscle. You might have also heard that it's 1–2 g per pound, but the body doesn't absorb that much protein and there's an increase in mortality rate with protein intake that high.

Protein is 4 calories per gram, carbohydrates are 4 calories per gram, and fat is 9 calories per gram.

You should consume about 30–40% of carbs an hour before your workout, and 30–40% of carbs immediately after. The remaining should be spread in the rest of the day.

Protein intake should be 0.6 grams per pound of bodyweight.

Fat intake should be 0.25–0.45 grams per pound of bodyweight.

Carb intake should be 1.25–1.5 grams per pound of bodyweight on training days. On rest days it should be about 0.5 grams per pound of bodyweight.

Why should protein intake be at 0.5–0.6 g/lb? The reason is that the increased mortality risk negates any benefits. Protein increases mortality rate by 400%.

HARRIS BENEDICT EQUATION FOR CALORIES CALCULATION

(10 x (POUNDS / 2.205)) + (6.25 x (INCHES x 2.54)) - ((5 x AGE) + 5)

Multiply the result by the coefficient depending on your activity level:

1.2 = Sedentary (no Activity)

1.375 = Lightly active (1–3 days/week)

1.55 = Moderately active (3–5 days/week)

1.725 = Very active (6–7 days/week)

1.9 = Extra active (very hard exercise or sports, and physically demanding job)

REPETITION MULTIPLIER TO CALCULATE APPROXIMATE MAX

1 REP = 100% OF WEIGHT

2 REPS = WEIGHT x 1.07

3 REPS = WEIGHT x 1.12

4 REPS = WEIGHT x 1.15

5 REPS = WEIGHT x 1.18

6 REPS = WEIGHT x 1.21

7 REPS = WEIGHT x 1.24

8 REPS = WEIGHT x 1.27

9 REPS = WEIGHT x 1.30

10 REPS = WEIGHT x 1.30

Add 0.03 to 1.12 per each additional rep. Do a failure set with a weight, then take the rep you failed at and multiply the weight by the number given to figure out your approximate one-rep maximum. If you've done your max, but want to figure out the reps for a lower weight, simply divide your max by the coefficient instead.

HITTING YOUR NUMBERS

Get in the habit of hitting your numbers. That means you should always strive to go up one more rep or hit the number of projected reps for a projected max.

SEQUENCES

The sequences are the most important part of this book. Without the sequences, this would just be an ordinary HIIT workout book. You are free to create your own sequences, however, I took the guesswork out of creating them. With these sequences you should be able to keep all sets to a minimum, which is one set.

For light to medium weight, the workhorse of the sequences will be the "forever sequence," named after myself, Bobby Forever. I know how brutal this sequence can be, and how much gains the forever sequence can produce. As a general rule of thumb for the forever sequence, use about 1/3 of the weight of your one-rep max to no more than 2/3 to 3/4 of your one-rep max.

For weight approaching your one-rep max use the partials sequence.

For exercises that are awkward, limited in range of motion, on a machine, or with a cable, use the pause sequence.

THE (BOBBY) FOREVER SEQUENCE

Begin with the prescribed repetitions. Next, do the lower third repetitions (the bottom third of the range of movement). Next, do the middle half repetitions (the middle of the range of movement). Next, do the upper third repetitions (the upper third of the range of movement). Next, do slow repetitions (full range of movement but slowly). Next, do a hold at the top third of the movement. Next, do a hold at the middle of the movement. Next, do a hold at the lower third of the movement. Lastly, hold halfway for a pre-determined time or until failure. All one sequence, all one set.

FOREVER SEQUENCE		
FULL REPS	: 7	PRESCRIBED REPS
1/3 REPS	: 7	
1/2 REPS	: 7	
2/3 REPS	: 7	
SLOW REPS	: 3	
1/3 PAUSE (sec)	: 3	
1/2 PAUSE (sec)	: 3	
2/3 PAUSE (sec)	: 3	
1/2 PAUSE (sec)	: 15 or failure	

FOREVER SEQUENCE TEMPLATE	
FULL REPS	:______________
1/3 REPS	:______________
1/2 REPS	:______________
2/3 REPS	:______________
SLOW REPS	:______________
1/3 PAUSE (sec)	:______________
1/2 PAUSE (sec)	:______________
2/3 PAUSE (sec)	:______________
1/2 PAUSE (sec)	:______________

PARTIALS SEQUENCE

Begin with the prescribed repetitions. Next, complete as many half-repetitions as possible. Next, complete as many quarter-repetitions as possible. If you still have some in the tank, complete a pause hold a quarter to a third of the way down, and if you still have some in the tank, complete some forced reps. Keep in mind that the majority of people will fail and gas out by the end of the quarter reps. However, you can take small ten-second breaks to keep going, if you want.

PARTIALS SEQUENCE		PARTIAL SEQUENCE TEMPLATE	
FULL REPS	: 6–20 PRESCRIBED REPS	FULL REPS	:________________
HALF REPS	: 3–10	HALF REPS	:________________
QUARTER REPS	: 1–5	QUARTER REPS	:________________
PAUSE/HOLD REP	: 1–15 sec	PAUSE/HOLD REP	:_____________sec
FORCED REPS	: 1–3	FORCED REPS	:________________

PAUSE SEQUENCE

Begin with the prescribed repetitions. Next, at the peak of the contraction hold for a time. Lastly, repeat as many times as possible. Note: you may adjust the pause time, where at in the range of motion you pause, and number of repetitions as you see fit.

PAUSE SEQUENCE		PAUSE SEQUENCE TEMPLATE	
FULL REPS	: 6–20 PRESCRIBED REPS	FULL REPS	:________________
PAUSE (sec)	: 3–10	PAUSE (sec)	:________________
REPEAT UNTIL FAILURE		REPEAT X TIMES or UNTIL FAILURE	

THE IDEAL MINIMALISTIC BODYBUILDING, POWERLIFTING, AND HIIT ROUTINE

ROUTINE #1 OR MONDAY (LEGS, TRAPS, CALVES, AND CORE)

(3 DAYS A WEEK)

SUMO SQUATS (ALT WITH REGULAR SQUAT)	1 x 6–20	TO FAILURE
ALTERNATE EVERY OTHER WEEK WITH SUMO DEADLIFTS (ALT WITH REGULAR DEADLIFTS)		
SHRUGS	1 x 12–20	PAUSE SEQUENCE
LEG-EXTENSIONS	1 x 12–20	FOREVER SEQUENCE
LEG-CURLS	1 x 12–20	FOREVER SEQUENCE
CALF-RAISES	1 x 12–20	PAUSE SEQUENCE OR FOREVER SEQ
CLEAN AND JERKS	1 x 1–10	MAY BE DONE AS FIRST EXERCISE
ABS	1 x 3–20	FOREVER SEQUENCE
SPRINT HIIT		

Of note here, sumo squats are done first, then sumo deadlifts the following Monday, then regular squats the following Monday, then regular deadlifts the following Monday. So, on a calendar, it would appear as follows:

1ST MONDAY: SUMO SQUATS

2ND MONDAY: SUMO DEADLIFTS

3RD MONDAY: REGULAR SQUATS

4TH MONDAY: REGULAR DEADLIFTS

SKIP HIIT, SKIP EXERCISES, SKIP WORKOUTS, ADJUST WEIGHT OR REPS AS NEEDED!

RECOVER, RECOVER, RECOVER!

THE IDEAL MINIMALISTIC BODYBUILDING, POWERLIFTING, AND HIIT ROUTINE

ROUTINE #2 OR WEDNESDAY (CHEST, SHOULDERS, AND TRICEPS)

(3 DAYS A WEEK)

BENCH-PRESS	1 x 3–10	PARTIALS SEQUENCE
ALT EVERY OTHER WEEK WITH INCLINE BENCH-PRESS		
DIPS	1 x 3–10	FOREVER SEQUENCE
OVERHEAD PRESS	1 x 6–12	PARTIALS OR FOREVER SEQUENCE
BARBELL TRICEPS-EXTENSIONS	1 x 6–12	PARTIALS OR FOREVER SEQUENCE
SNATCH	1 x 1–10	MAY BE DONE AS FIRST EXERCISE
BURPEES HIIT		

SKIP HIIT, SKIP EXERCISES, SKIP WORKOUTS, ADJUST WEIGHT OR REPS AS NEEDED!

RECOVER, RECOVER, RECOVER!

THE IDEAL MINIMALISTIC BODYBUILDING, POWERLIFTING, AND HIIT ROUTINE

ROUTINE #3 OR FRIDAY (BACK, MID-BACK, BICEPS, AND FOREARMS)

(3 DAYS A WEEK)

PULL-UPS	1 x 3–12	FOREVER OR PARTIALS SEQUENCE
ALT EVERY OTHER WEEK WITH CHIN-UPS		
BENT-OVER-ROWS W/REV. FLYS	1 x 3–12	FOREVER OR PAUSE SEQUENCE
BARBELL CURLS W/WRIST CURLS	1 x 3–12	FOREVER OR PAUSE SEQUENCE
SHADOWBOXING HIIT		

SKIP HIIT, SKIP EXERCISES, SKIP WORKOUTS, ADJUST WEIGHT OR REPS AS NEEDED!

RECOVER, RECOVER, RECOVER!

ROUTINE #1 EXECUTION

This is our Monday, and it's our first legs workout. So, from our repetition multiplier we've figured out the weight needed to do the prescribed reps.

SUMO SQUATS (LEGS)

First of all, you and your spotter do the proper warm-up of at least two sets. The first set at 50% of your target weight, for no more than 10 reps. The second set at 75% of your target weight, for no more than 5 reps. Now, for the working set, the set that has the target weight loaded up with. Begin by un-racking the weight on the meaty part of your traps and shoulders. Next, spread your legs out as much as possible, while still allowing you to squat to a parallel squat, with your thighs parallel to the ground. Next, bend at the knees, as if you are taking an imaginary seat. Squat without tilting forward, and make sure to look up or at least not down. Lastly, stand back up. Commence the prescribed repetitions until failure or following a sequence.

ALT EVERY OTHER WEEK WITH SUMO DEADLIFTS (LEGS AND WHOLE BODY)

You will only squat once a week, or deadlift once a week, but not both in the same week. If both deadlift and squat are done in the same week, it can quickly lead to central nervous system fatigue or overtraining.

First of all, you and your spotter do the proper warmup of at least two sets. The first set at 50% of your target weight, for no more than 10 reps. The second set at 75% of your target weight, for no more than 5 reps. Now, for the working set, the set that has the target weight loaded up with. Begin by assuming the sumo deadlift position, feet spread across, much like the bottom position of a sumo squat, as if you're semi-seated. Hand running down on the inside of your legs, not the outside. Next, you simply stand up straight. Commence the prescribed repetitions until failure or the appropriate sequence.

SHRUGS (TRAPS)

Begin by holding the bar in front of you at about the waist, arms hanging naturally but not relaxed. Next, keeping your arms straight and elbows locked out, bring your shoulders up towards your ears. It would appear as if you're trying to say, "I don't know" with your body language. Once the prescribed repetitions are completed, commence the Pause sequence or the appropriate sequence.

LEG-EXTENSIONS (QUADS)

Begin seated with your shins against the padding of the machine. Next, extend your legs out until the knee is fully locked out. Once the prescribed repetitions are completed, commence the Forever sequence or the appropriate sequence.

LEG-CURLS (HAMSTRINGS)

Begin by lying face-down, or standing up against your machine, depending on your equipment. Next, bring your ankles toward your butt. Once the prescribed repetitions are completed, commence the Forever sequence or the appropriate sequence.

CALF-RAISES (CALVES)

Begin with a barbell on your back as if you're about to squat. Next, raise your heels up as if standing on your tippy toes. Once the prescribed repetitions are completed, commence the pause sequence.

CLEAN AND JERK (WHOLE BODY)

A Clean implies a full squat. Begin by grasping shoulder-width apart, palms facing down a barbell on the ground. You should stand with legs shoulder-width apart, with knees bent in a semi-seated position. Next, come up with the bar as if doing a regular deadlift, not a sumo deadlift. Simultaneously use your calves, but do not lift your toes off the ground. Once the bar is above waist level, drop to a full squat, that's ass-to-calves. Next, catch the bar. It would appear as if you're in the bottom position of a front squat. Next, stand up.

Next, Jerk the bar above your head. That is to say dip at the knees as if doing a push-press and explode the bar up above your head. Depending on whether you're left foot dominant or right foot dominant, it will dictate which leg will be in front of you, and which leg will be behind you. It would appear as if you push-pressed with your knees bent, one leg in front of you, the other behind. Lastly, at this point recover your foot placement, and bring the bar down to the floor. Commence the set.

ABS

There are many options out there, and the decline bench sit-ups will be our main focus. Decline bench sit-ups are simply sit-ups you do on a decline bench. Begin by lying on the decline bench with feet locked in and arms across your chest. Next, make your upper torso come up by hinging forward at the waist, until sitting straight up. Once the prescribed repetitions are completed, commence the forever sequence.

SPRINT HIIT

Sprint on a track for 10–15 seconds, or some designated portion of it. Next, jog slow for about 30–60 seconds, or some designated portion of the track, as a means of recovering. On the recovery portion you can never go too slow. Next, pick up the pace by running 15–30 seconds, or some designated portion of the track. At this portion your speed should be faster than your recovery jog, but slower than your sprint speed. Complete this at least 3 to 5 times, for no more than 15–20 minutes.

ROUTINE #2 EXECUTION

This is our Wednesday, and it's our first chest workout. So, from our repetition multiplier we've figured out the weight needed to do the prescribed reps.

BENCH-PRESS (CHEST, TRICEPS, AND SHOULDERS)

First of all, you and your spotter do the proper warmup of at least two sets. The first set at 50% of your target weight, for no more than 10 repetitions. The second set at 75% of your target weight, for no more than 5 repetitions. Now, for the working set, the set that has the target weight loaded up on it. Begin by getting in the proper position, that is feet firmly planted on the ground with your back arched. Next, un-rack the weight with hands more than shoulder-width apart. Next, lower the weight until the bar touches your chest or at least the upper torso. Push the weight up, digging your feet in the ground, driving through the quads. Once the prescribed repetitions are completed, commence the Partials sequence or the appropriate sequence.

ALT EVERY OTHER WEEK WITH INCLINE BENCH-PRESS (UPPER CHEST, SHOULDERS, TRICEPS)

Incline bench-press is the same exercise, with the bench angled upward. Don't go too crazy on the angle as a 30–45-degree angle is all that is needed. All that was said of the regular bench-press still applies here. Once the prescribed repetitions are completed, commence the Partials sequence or the appropriate sequence.

DIPS (LOWER CHEST, SHOULDERS, AND TRICEPS)

Dips may be done with either your bodyweight, weighted, or even assisted if needed. Begin by holding the dip bars until suspended in mid-air. From an arms-locked-out position, descend down until a nice comfortable stretch is achieved across the chest. Lastly, push yourself back up. Once the prescribed repetitions are completed, commence the Forever sequence or the appropriate sequence.

OVERHEAD PRESS (SHOULDERS AND TRICEPS)

Begin by holding the barbell with your hands a little more than shoulder-width apart, above chest level. Next, press the weight upwards until your arms are fully extended. Lastly, lower the weight. Once the prescribed repetitions are completed, commence the Forever sequence or the appropriate sequence.

BARBELL TRICEPS-EXTENSIONS (TRICEPS)

Begin by holding the barbell overhead, with your hands less than a shoulder-width apart. Next, bend your elbows so that your forearm goes behind your head and your elbows stay pointed upward. Lastly, extend your arms out so that the weight is back over your head. Once the prescribed repetitions are completed, commence the Forever sequence or appropriate sequence.

SNATCH (WHOLE BODY)

To snatch implies to do a full squat. Begin by standing in front of a barbell on the ground, feet either shoulder-width apart or more. Hold the barbell with palms facing down as far apart as possible, for most bars and people it is hands outside the outer rings. Next, from a seated position, lift the weight upward as if doing a deadlift, raising your heels but not your toes, as far as possible. Next, once the weight is above waist level, begin raising the bar up with elbows as straight as possible. Simultaneously, drop to a full squat as you raise the bar above your head. It would appear as if you are at the bottom of a full squat (ass-to-calves) holding a barbell over your head. Next, with arms locked out, stand up. Lastly, bring the barbell back to the floor. Commence the set.

BURPEES HIIT

Do about 1 minute of burpees. Next, do 30 seconds of jumping jacks. Lastly, jog a lap or jog in place. Complete this at least 3 to 5 times, for no more than 15–20 minutes.

ROUTINE #3 EXECUTION

This is our Friday, and it's our first back workout. So, from our repetition multiplier we've figured out the weight needed to do the prescribed repetitions.

PULL-UPS (LATS, BACK, BICEPS, AND FOREARMS)

The pull-ups may be done with either bodyweight, weighted, or even assisted. Begin by doing a couple of warm-up sets. Hold onto the pull-up bar with hands shoulder-width apart, palms facing away from you. Next, pull yourself up all the way. Lastly, lower yourself. Once the prescribed repetitions are completed, commence the Forever sequence or the appropriate sequence.

ALT EVERY OTHER WEEK WITH CHIN-UPS (LATS, BACK, BICEPS, AND FOREARMS)

Chin-ups are performed just like pull-ups, except with palms facing towards you.

BENT-OVER ROWS (MID-BACK, BICEPS, FOREARMS)

Begin by standing in front of the barbell, with feet shoulder-width apart. Pick-up the barbell and hold it with your elbows straight. Hinge at the waist forward, for about 45 degrees. Next, pull the barbell towards your stomach. Lastly, lower the weight while maintaining your body at a 45-degree angle. Once the prescribed repetitions are completed, commence the forever sequence.

DUMBBELL REVERSE FLYS (MID-BACK, REAR-SHOULDER)

Begin by standing with a pair of dumbbells in your hands. Next, hinge forward at the hips, for about 45 degrees. Next, with elbows as straight as possible, move the dumbbells upward, palms facing down. It would appear as if you're flapping your arms. Lastly, bring the dumbbells back down, your whole movement under control. Once the prescribed repetitions are completed, commence the pause sequence or the appropriate sequence.

BARBELL CURLS (BICEPS AND FOREARMS)

Begin by standing, holding a barbell, hands shoulder-width apart. Next, keeping your back straight, and elbows locked into your sides, lift the barbell upward toward your chest. Lastly, bring the weight back down, your whole movement under control. Once the prescribed repetitions are completed, commence the Forever sequence or the appropriate sequence.

WRIST CURLS (FOREARMS)

Begin by sitting on a bench holding a barbell overhanging past your knees, with elbows locked on top of your legs. Next, let the wrist naturally hinge down to where the barbell is along your knees. Next, using only your wrists, lift the weight up. Lastly, bring the weight back down, under control. Once the prescribed repetitions are completed, commence the Pause sequence or the appropriate sequence.

SHADOWBOXING HIIT

Shadowbox, throwing punch combinations for 30–60 seconds. Next, start doing footwork for 30–60 seconds focusing on dodging imaginary punches from an imaginary opponent. Lastly, jog a lap or jog in place. Repeat at least 3 to 5 times, for no more than 15–20 minutes.

THE MINIMALISTIC ROUTINE

(3 DAYS A WEEK OR EVEN 3 DAYS EVERY TWO WEEKS)

ROUTINE #1 OR MONDAY TOTAL-BODY WORKOUT

REGULAR SQUATS OR SUMO SQUATS	1 x 3–12	NO SEQUENCE
REGULAR BENCH-PRESS OR INCLINE BENCH-PRESS	1 x 3–12	NO SEQUENCE
REGULAR DEADLIFTS OR SUMO DEADLIFTS	1 x 3–12	NO SEQUENCE
PULL-UPS OR CHIN-UPS	1 x 3–12	NO SEQUENCE
AB-ROLLER	1 x 3–12	NO SEQUENCE

ROUTINE #2 OR WEDNESDAY OLYMPIC LIFTS

MAY BE SWITCHED WITH ROUTINE #1

CLEAN AND JERKS	1 x 3–12
ALT EVERY OTHER WEEK WITH THE SNATCH	1 x 3–12

ROUTINE #3 OR FRIDAY HIIT DAY

HIIT	1 x FOR NO MORE THAN 5 MINUTES

Do not doubt the efficacy of this training routine as it is what in HIIT we call a consolidated routine. An all-lean routine with no fat.

THE IDEAL MINIMALISTIC SINGLE WORKOUT ROUTINE

CLEAN AND JERK	1 x FAILURE
SNATCH	1 x FAILURE
INCLINE BENCH-PRESS	1 x FAILURE SEQUENCE OR NOT
PULL-UPS	1 x FAILURE SEQUENCE OR NOT
REGULAR OR SUMO SQUAT	1 x FAILURE SEQUENCE OR NOT
REGULAR OR SUMO DEADLIFT	1 x FAILURE SEQUENCE OR NOT
OVERHEAD PRESS	1 x FAILURE SEQUENCE OR NOT
BARBELL ROW	1 x FAILURE SEQUENCE OR NOT
SHRUGS	1 x FAILURE SEQUENCE OR NOT
BARBELL CURLS	1 x FAILURE SEQUENCE OR NOT
BARBELL TRICEPS-EXTENSION	1 x FAILURE SEQUENCE OR NOT
BARBELL WRIST CURLS	1 x FAILURE SEQUENCE OR NOT
CALF RAISES	1 x FAILURE SEQUENCE OR NOT
ABS	1 x FAILURE SEQUENCE OR NOT
HIIT	1 x FOR NO MORE THAN 15 MIN

THE IDEAL MINIMALISTIC BODYBUILDING ROUTINE

BENCH-PRESS	1 x 3–12	SEQUENCE
ALT EVERY OTHER WEEK WITH INCLINE BENCH-PRESS		
OVERHEAD PRESS	1 x 6–12	SEQUENCE
PULL-UP	1 x 6–12	SEQUENCE
ALT EVERY OTHER WEEK WITH CHIN-UP		
BENT-OVER ROW	1 x 6–12	SEQUENCE
FULL SQUAT	1 x 6–20	SEQUENCE
ALT EVERY OTHER WEEK WITH REGULAR DEADLIFT		
CALF-RAISES	1 x 6–20	SEQUENCE
ABS	1 x 6–20	SEQUENCE
BARBELL CURLS	1 x 6–12	SEQUENCE
BARBELL TRICEPS-EXTENSION	1 x 6–12	SEQUENCE

FULL SQUAT (THIGHS AND LOWER BACK)

Begin by un-racking a barbell onto the meaty part of your traps and shoulders, standing with feet shoulder-width apart. Next, bend at the knees until your calves stop you from going down further. It would appear as if you're sitting on an imaginary stool. Make sure to keep your back straight throughout the entire movement. Lastly, stand back up.

REGULAR DEADLIFT (WHOLE BODY)

Begin by standing with feet shoulder-width apart in front of a barbell on the ground. Next, grasp the barbell with both palms facing away from you, with hands wider than shoulder-width apart. Lastly, from a semi seated position, with your back straight, stand up.

TOTAL BODY HOLE-SHOT WORKOUT ROUTINE

REGULAR PUSH-UP OR DEEP PUSH-UP	1 x 6–12	SEQUENCE
REGULAR SQUAT OR PISTOL SQUAT	1 x 12–20	SEQUENCE
LAT FLEXES	1 x 15–60 SECONDS	REPEAT
BODY PRESS OR HANDSTAND PUSH-UP	1 x 6–12	SEQUENCE
BICEP FLEXES	1 x 15–60 SECONDS	REPEAT
CHINESE PUSH-UP OR DIPS	1 x 6–12	SEQUENCE
SIT-UPS OR FLAGS	1 x 12–20	SEQUENCE
QUAD FLEXES	1 x 15–60 SECONDS	REPEAT
SINGLE LEG STRAIGHT LEG DEADLIFT	1 x 12–20	SEQUENCE
CALF RAISES OR SINGLE LEG CALF RAISE	1 x 12–20	SEQUENCE
INVERTED-ROW	1 x 6–12	SEQUENCE
TRAP FLEXES	1 x 15–60 SECONDS	REPEAT

You're going to wish you had weightlifting equipment, because if done correctly, the Hole-Shot workout is intense to say the least. Notice that now the introduction of flexing is included. Flexing is now an exercise, and don't underestimate it, as it's intense and will enlarge the muscle, if done correctly and sufficiently.

REGULAR PUSH-UP (CHEST, SHOULDERS, AND TRICEPS)

Begin by lying face-down prone, feet shoulder-width apart, and hands more than shoulder-width apart. Make sure your weight is sustained on your hands, with elbows locked-out. Next, descend by bending at the elbows. Lastly, once your chest touches the ground, press yourself up. Once the prescribed reps are completed, commence the appropriate sequence.

DEEP PUSH-UP (CHEST, SHOULDERS, AND TRICEPS)

Deep push-ups are performed just like regular push-ups, except with hands elevated by something, such as books. Feet may also be elevated. Once the prescribed reps are completed, commence the appropriate sequence.

REGULAR SQUAT (THIGHS)

Begin by standing with feet shoulder-width apart. Next, bend at the knees until you are down in a full squat. Lastly, stand up. Once the prescribed reps are completed, commence the appropriate sequence.

PISTOL SQUAT (THIGH)

Essentially a one-legged squat. Begin by standing on one leg, and balance yourself with your hands in front of you. Next, bend at the knee until all the way down. Lastly, stand up, using your arms to balance your weight. Once the prescribed reps are completed, commence the appropriate sequence.

LAT FLEXES (LATS)

This exercise requires body control. Begin by placing your hands to your side, making a fist, with elbows pointed out. Next, flex your lats for the prescribed amount of time. Next, release, breathing adequately enough to catch your breath. Lastly, commence flexing again. Flexes are the only exercise that will be repeated until sore.

BODY PRESS (SHOULDERS AND TRICEPS)

Begin by standing with legs shoulder-width apart. Next, hinge at the waist forward until your hands touch the ground, with hands shoulder-width apart. It would appear as if you're making an upside-down U with the ground. Next, bend at the elbows, until your head comes close to touching the ground, but not hitting the ground. Lastly, press yourself up by straightening out your elbows. Once the prescribed reps are complete, commence the appropriate sequence.

HANDSTAND PUSH-UP (SHOULDERS, TRICEPS, AND TRAPS)

These can be done against a wall or free-standing. Begin by standing on your hands. Next, bend at the elbows until your head comes close to touching the ground, but not hitting the ground. Lastly, press yourself up, by straightening out your elbows. Once the prescribed reps have been completed, commence the appropriate sequence.

BICEP FLEXES (BICEPS)

Begin by flexing both biceps as if you're looking at yourself in the mirror and checking out your gains, with elbows pointed away from your sides for the prescribed amount of time. Lastly, release. Once you've caught your breath, repeat as many times as necessary until sore.

CHINESE PUSH-UP

Chinese push-ups are much like body presses, except with hands close together, less than shoulder-width apart. Once the prescribed reps are completed, commence the appropriate sequence.

DIPS (CHEST, SHOULDERS, AND TRICEPS)

If your cell has a table, you can do dips. Begin by facing away from the table, with the meaty part of your palms on the table's edge. Next, place your legs away from you so that all of your weight is supported by your palms. Next, dip down by bending at the elbows. Lastly, press-up by straightening your elbows. Once the prescribed reps have been completed, commence the appropriate sequence.

INVERTED ROW (MIDDLE BACK AND BICEPS)

If your cell has a table, you can do inverted rows. Begin by sitting under your table. Next, grab the end of your table with your hands. Next, straighten out your body. It would appear as if you are making a slanted I with the table. Lastly, pull yourself up to the table. Once the prescribed reps have been completed, commence the appropriate sequence.

TRAP FLEXES (TRAPS)

Begin by flexing your traps as if doing the most muscular pose you can, for the prescribed amount of time. Lastly, release. Once you've caught your breath repeat until you are sore.

SIT-UPS (ABDOMINALS)

Begin by lying prone on the ground, face up, with a bend in the knees, and feet secured under something. Next, hinge at the waist until your upper torso meets your thighs. For most, it is usually elbows touching the knees. Lastly, descend in a controlled manner. Once the prescribed repetitions are completed, commence the appropriate sequence.

FLAGS (ABDOMINALS)

Begin by lying prone on the ground, face up, holding onto something with your hands. Next, raise your legs up. Next, raise your hips off the ground. It would appear as if you are on the ground with just your upper back and neck area making contact with the ground and with your legs in the air. Lastly, lower your legs back down in a controlled manner. Once the prescribed reps are completed, commence the appropriate sequence.

QUAD FLEXES (QUADS)

Begin by flexing your quads for the prescribed amount of time. Lastly, release, once you've caught your breath. Repeat as many times as necessary until sore. Once the prescribed reps are complete, commence the appropriate sequence.

SINGLE LEG STRAIGHT LEG DEADLIFT (HAMSTRINGS)

Begin by standing straight. Next, standing on one leg, hinge at the hips until there is a muscular stretch on the hamstring and glutes of the leg you are standing on. Lastly, return to standing position. Once the prescribed repetitions are completed, commence the appropriate sequence. Complete for each leg.

CALF-RAISES (CALVES)

Begin by standing straight. Next, elevate your heels while keeping your toes on the ground. It would appear as if you are standing on your tippy toes. Lastly descend in a controlled manner. Once the prescribed reps are completed, commence the appropriate sequence.

SINGLE LEG CALF-RAISES (CALVES)

Single leg calf-raises are done one leg at a time.

SPLIT FOR 7 DAYS A WEEK

SUNDAY	:	CHEST, SHOULDERS
MONDAY	:	TRICEPS, SHINS (OPTIONAL)
TUESDAY	:	LATS, MIDDLE BACK
WEDNESDAY	:	BICEPS, FOREARMS
THURSDAY	:	LEGS, CALVES
FRIDAY	:	ABS
SATURDAY	:	CLEAN AND JERK, SNATCH

SPLIT FOR 2 DAYS A WEEK

1) UPPER BODY

2) LOWER BODY, OLYMPIC LIFTS

SPLIT FOR 3 DAYS A WEEK

1) PUSH

2) PULL

3) LEGS, OLYMPIC LIFTS

SPLIT FOR 4 DAYS A WEEK

1) PUSH OVERHEAD

2) PUSH STRAIGHT

3) PULL

4) LEGS, OLYMPIC LIFTS

SPLIT FOR 5 DAYS A WEEK

1) PUSH OVERHEAD

2) PUSH STRAIGHT

3) PULL

4) BICEPS AND TRICEPS

5) LEGS, OLYMPIC LIFTS

SPLIT FOR 6 DAYS A WEEK

1) PUSH OVERHEAD

2) PUSH STRAIGHT

3) PULL STRAIGHT

4) PULL DOWNWARD

5) BICEPS AND TRICEPS

6) LEGS, OLYMPIC LIFTS

NECK

Neck will usually not be a problem, except for some it is.

A neck brace is a piece of equipment that can be used to support the neck. However, there are bodyweight and other exercises for strengthening it.

Neck planks; front, back, and side.

Neck crunches; lying front, lying back, lying sideways.

HIIT ONLY

Undoubtedly, there are going to be those of you who either don't want to or are tired of bodybuilding and powerlifting workouts. For those of you that want a HIIT-only way of working out, these next routines are for you.

WHAT IS HIIT

Work involving brief intervals of high intensity exercise alternated with low intensity exercise. Repeated for a total of only minutes of exercise. In other words, peaks and valleys of activity.

THE 7-MINUTE WORKOUT

Designed by exercise physiologists at the Human Performance Institute, it includes twelve exercises. You do the exercises as many times as you can in 30 seconds, then you give yourself a 5 second break, until you get through all 12 exercises.

90% of MAX HEART RATE

MAX HEART RATE = 220 – AGE

1) JUMPING JACKS

2) WALL SITS

3) PUSH-UPS

4) AB CRUNCHES

5) STEP UPS

6) SQUATS

7) TRICEPS DIPS

8) PLANKS

9) HIGH KNEES

10) LUNGES

11) PUSH-UP ROTATION

12) SIDE PLANKS

EPOC

Excess Post-Exercise Oxygen Consumption: Often called afterburn. The excess oxygen burns up fat at an increased rate after the workout. Said to be for up to 48 hours. EPOC is triggered more by the intensity of a workout than by the duration of a workout.

HGH

Once the fast twitch fibers are activated, the body releases HGH, the Human Growth Hormone, said to be as high as 700 percent.

CORTISOL

Cortisol starts to appear after 20 minutes of "cardio," and 45–60 minutes of "working out." Cortisol is a stress hormone that competes with Testosterone. Cortisol is bad, as it promotes muscle break-down and fat retention in the stomach.

THE ADVANCED 7-MINUTE WORKOUT

1) REVERSE LUNGE; ELBOW TO INSTEP WITH ROTATION, ALTERNATING SIDES; 30 SECONDS

2) LATERAL PILLAR BRIDGE (LEFT); 30 SECONDS

3) PUSH-UP TO ROW TO BURPEE; 60 SECONDS

4) LATERAL PILLAR BRIDGE (RIGHT); 30 SECONDS

5) SINGLE-LEG ROMANIAN DEADLIFT TO CURL TO PRESS; 30 SECONDS EACH SIDE

6) PLANK WITH ARM LIFT; 30 SECONDS

7) LATERAL LUNGE TO OVERHEAD TRICEPS-EXTENSION; 60 SECONDS

8) BENT OVER ROW; 60 SECONDS

PART TWO

NUTS AND BOLTS

PHILOSOPHY

Minimal wear and tear: Part of the high-intensity philosophy is to induce the least possible taxing wear and tear on the body. This also reduces the occurrence of repetitive stress injuries.

The point is that the body only has so much that it can take in terms of wear and tear. So, exercise minimally to yield the largest amount of gains possible.

THE MINDSET

MAX INTENSITY, MAX RECOVERY, FOR MAX GAINS

"Workout intensely, infrequently, and when not, be in recovery."

"Workout intensely" by using as many of the high-intensity techniques and practices possible in practicality.

"Infrequently," once a week or less stimulation to the body is all that is needed. Not only for sufficient gains but efficient gains as well. Remember, exercise is a catabolic (breaking down) stimulus that triggers an anabolic (building) effect. After exercise, you get weaker, not stronger. Strength only comes after you've recovered, which may be 4 to 7 days or even 10, 14, to even 21 days, depending on the individual and how advanced they are.

"Be in recovery," pretty much anything that is not taxing the body or as long as it's a eustress (a positive stressor) on the body.

This follows the minimalistic mindset: "Do the least to get the most."

"Do the least" entails the least amount of sets, reps, rest, exercises, load, etc.; you get the idea. This is different for everyone.

"To get the most," entails you getting the most bang for your buck, so to speak. If one set to failure makes you grow in a measurable way either by strength, number of reps, or size, then, that's all you need. I don't know how many times people say, "I'm already sore," and yet they keep going. Remember, more is not best. You will get diminishing returns really quick.

STIMULI/EXERCISE

A stimulus is something that brings about a certain action or response.

Exercise is a stimulus and the sets and reps of an exercise are the means of this stimulus

The response we are obviously looking for from exercise is to become more anabolically fit and anaerobically fit as well.

ONE SET RESEARCH

So, remember, we are only concerned with setting in motion the growth mechanism and leaving it alone. Regarding HIIT, we are only concerned with setting in motion EPOC and leaving it alone.

Remember, exercise is a catabolic stimulus; you get weaker after exercise, not stronger.

ONE SET

You only need to activate the body's growth mechanism once via exercise. *There is no need to constantly activate the growth mechanism via multiple sets.* Therefore, only one set is all that is needed. One set to failure and beyond.

For the majority of you, this will be one set unlike anything you've ever done.

WAYS IN WHICH TO GET YOU TO ONE SET OF SEQUENCES

1 ¼ REPS, 1/3 REPS, 1 ½ REPS, ½ REPS, 1 ¾ REPS, ¾ REPS, etc...

PAUSE REPS SET: Where you pause somewhere in the rep, for time or failure.

PYRAMID REP SET: 1 REP, ¼ REP, ½ REP, ¾ REP, BACK TO 1 REP.

21S 7 FULL REPS — 7 LOWER HALF REPS — 7 UPPER HALF REPS

WAYS IN WHICH TO GET TO ONE SET

10 sets of 10; down to "10 UP" or "10 DOWN." 10 UP is when you start with 1 and go up 1 rep a set until 10, and 10 DOWN is when you start with 10 and go down 1 rep a set until you reach 1.

6 SETS OF 6 OR 6 SETS OF 5

5 SETS OF 5 OR 5 SETS OF 6

3 SETS OF 1–3 OR 4–6 OR 7–10

2 SETS OF 1–5 OR 6–10

1 SET OF SEQUENCE

Note: 1 set of a "burnout" is basically a huge dropset.

HIGH INTENSITY TECHNIQUES

TRAINING TO FAILURE: Another rep is not possible.

PRE-EXHAUSTION: Exhaust a muscle or muscle groups.

PEAK CONTRACTION: Contract and hold at the peak of the movement.

FORCED REPS: With a spotter, force reps out.

NEGATIVE REPS: Bring a weight down (usually slowly, but under control).

REST-PAUSE: Pause long enough, before muscles recover. Usually for 10 seconds.

PARTIAL REPS: Limit the range of movement.

STATIC CONTRACTION: Hold the weight still. Usually for 3 or more seconds.

SPOTTER-APPLIED RESISTANCE: The spotter pushes down on the weight.

MULTISET: 2 or more exercises back-to-back, including supersets.

SEQUENCE: Chaining one high-intensity technique after another.

MINI-SET: Spurts of reps, where it is acceptable to temporarily rack the weight.

MICRO-SET: Do not rack the weight, while doing spurts of reps.

BEYOND FAILURE: Reaching failure then resting just enough to keep going.

DROPSET: Lower the weight to continue the set, including burnouts.

BILATERAL DEFICIT

A bilateral deficit is the lack of contraction capability of one muscle compared to another. Bilateral deficit is the reason so many will find it difficult to get biceps the same size, as well as other body parts.

OXYGEN DEFICIT

Oxygen deficit occurs when the muscle's oxygen demand can't be met. Therefore, many will find that they may terminate a set early, not because they can't keep lifting, but because they can't catch their breath. The best way to deal with this is to pause the set and breathe for 10 seconds, then resume. Keep doing this technique as you see fit.

OVERSTIMULATION

Overstimulation can easily creep up, just like overtraining, since once the growth mechanism has been activated, it will be interrupted by another stimulus, that is by other exercise. The easiest and best way to deal with this problem is to do away with the excess stimulation. Another but less effective way is to limit the overstimulation to the same workout.

OVERTRAINING

In an attempt to get big and lean, most people will overtrain under the false thinking that "more is better."

OVERTRAINING CHECKBOX

___ TAKES A LONG TIME TO WARM UP

___ PLATEAUING

___ LOSS OF STRENGTH

___ ELEVATED HEART RATE

___ FATIGUE DURING THE DAY

___ EARLY EXHAUSTION DURING A WORKOUT AKA "GASSING OUT"

___ LOSS OF APPETITE

___ DISTURBED DIGESTION

___ MENTAL DULLNESS AKA "LOSS OF MOTIVATION"

___ WEIGHT LOSS

___ INJURY

RECOVERY

Recovery is something everyone agrees that's important, but few agree on what it is.

Bar none, the single most important recovery is sleep. This not only is *vital* to the human race but is almost exclusively the way the body produces the Human Growth Hormone (HGH), a vital hormone to gains and wellness.

Some other ways to recover are through stretching, foam rolling, icing, hot baths or showers, and massages.

ACTIVE RECOVERY

Active recovery refers to being physically active in some way, without exhausting previously worked muscles. This method isn't completely set in stone, it's up to you the individual. Just note, be mindful of what can quickly become overtraining and cut into your overall recovery, and consecutively, gains.

HYDRATION

Muscles are composed of about 75–80% water. Being properly hydrated maximizes your circulation blood volume, which in turn maximizes the number of nutrients that reach the muscles, all the while discarding waste products that arise.

MUSCLE FIBERS

MOTOR UNITS: Consist of muscle fibers that are all the same type. The so-called fast, intermediate, and slow twitch.

ALL OR NONE LAW: When a motor unit is activated, all of its muscle fibers are activated.

SEQUENTIAL RECRUITMENT: Motor units can contract sequentially, such as when lower order muscle fibers fatigue and are replaced by higher order muscle fibers.

Slow twitch motor units contain about 100 muscle fibers.

Fast twitch motor units contain about 10,000 muscle fibers.

Should take about a minute to a minute and a half to exhaust the motor units collectively.

Fast twitch motor units can take 4 to 10 days to recover, or even longer at times.

Slow twitch motor units are readily available after a rest of about 90 seconds.

MUSCLE CONTRACTIONS

Typically, the maximum possible percentage of total muscle fibers that can contract at any given moment is about 30 percent.

THE 3 WAYS A MUSCLE CONTRACTS

POSITIVE or CONCENTRIC where the muscle shortens.

NEGATIVE or ECCENTRIC where the muscle lengthens.

STATIC or ISOMETRIC where the muscle is being used, but doesn't lengthen or shorten, and instead stays in place.

THE (BOBBY) FOREVER PROGRESSION SYSTEM

Without a doubt, one of the most important systems you will need in the beginning is a progression type system. The easiest system is the one I use, where you just work towards the end of a rep range, before increasing the weight for about 20 pounds.

This works for two reasons. First, the weight increase should put you back down to the beginning of the rep range. Second, the prison I was at only allowed for the most part 20 lb. increments.

For example: On legs, I like to go for 6 reps. So, 6 reps could either be the beginning or the end of the rep range, either way I go for a 3-rep range. So, if 6 is the end of my rep range, I subtract 3, for a 3–6 rep range, which would mean that I'm going rather heavy. Now, if I don't want to go that heavy, I add 3 reps to 6 for a total of 9. So, the rep range would be 6–9. This makes a huge difference and allows me to experiment with different weights.

At the time of writing, my full-squat, aka bucket squat, was 335 pounds. If I wanted to go heavy and work my way up, I'd start with a weight of 315 pounds for 3 reps and work my way up one rep at a time per workout until I'm at 6 reps, before adding a dime on each side, bringing the weight up to 335 pounds for 3 reps, then doing it all over again. Now, if I wanted to go lighter, I'd start with 6 reps of about 295 pounds and work my way up to 9 reps, until finally adding a dime on each side and repeating the process all over again.

A SIMPLE CHART OF THE FOREVER PROGRESSION SYSTEM

3 reps	9 reps	16 reps	AND SO ON...
1–3 or 3–6	6–9 or 9–12	12–16 or 16–20	

As strength is the primary attribute I go for, I use 3 and 9 the most while occasionally using 16 or more when a de-load is in order, or when trying to increase muscle size and joint strength. No matter what though, one thing should always remain, and that is the use of low sets; preferably a single one.

SKIPPING EXERCISES: SKIP SMARTLY

In order to prevent injury and overtraining, skipping exercises is a great way to keep going.

For example, the prior week was deadlifts and now you have squats. However, your lower back is tender from the deadlifts. Well, skip squats for the week, give your lower back that extra week to recover. Sometimes, it can be a simple matter of splitting your routine. For instance, one week you had sumo squats, but your energy levels were all used up. So, you do half the routine which was sumo squats and calf raises but completed the abs and traps later on that day or even the next day. Also, your hip extensors were feeling a bit over-taxed, so you skipped lunges, as normally you pair that with laps to get a HIIT workout.

Point is, I see people constantly injure themselves and keep themselves from recovering, just because they simply didn't listen to their body.

Now, that doesn't mean I hate certain exercises, therefore I'm going to skip those exercises. Nope, do especially the exercises you least enjoy.

PERIODIZATION

PERIODIZATION: A planned-out period of working out.

LINEAR: You move through weight and rep schemes linearly.

UNDULATING: You move through weight and rep schemes in a wavelike form.

BLOCK: 3 phases of 4–8 weeks; first phase at 55–75%, second at 75–90%, third at 90% or more.

CONJUGATE: You move through weight and rep schemes that increase hypertrophy, absolute strength, and dynamic strength. For hypertrophy, you deal in high reps, of about 9 or more. For absolute strength, you deal in low reps, at about the 3 range. And for dynamic strength, you deal in weight that allows you to lift with speed in mind, usually 2–3 seconds for 2–3 reps.

STICKING POINTS

Sticking points is when and where in the movement you get stuck at. As an example, you might have moved the weight almost through the entire range of motion, however, you can't move it past a certain point. This will be different for every lift. Most commonly for the bench-press, it's in the lower-middle of the movement, while some people may get stuck at the lock-out portion of the lift.

The culprit behind sticking points is actually quite simple. It's due to something known as "moment arm." "Moment arm" is when and where the joint is at its most horizontal, moving into and out of moment arm is typically the sticking point.

It's actually a Physics term. I could've bored you with a bunch of math and show off how smart I am, or I can just tell you what you need to know about it. I choose the latter. But, basically, it's the sticking point since all the possible muscle fibers have to contract, to keep holding or moving the weight. Not to be confused with the peak of the contraction.

THE (BOBBY) FOREVER PERIODIZATION SYSTEM

CREATING A PERIODIZATION TABLE

Using the repetition multiplier, figure out the weight and reps as you increase steadily by a week or so.

For instance, suppose I'm going from a 295-pound bench-press max to a 315-pound bench-press max. Our increment a week will be 5 pounds and our repetitions will be undulating (waveform). So, our table will look like this.

WEEK	WEIGHT x REPS	PROJECTED MAX
1	295 x 1	295
2	267 x 3	300
3	258 x 5	305
4	276 x 3	310
5	315 x 1	315

VALSALVA MANEUVER ON MAXIMAL LIFTS

Holding your breath while doing an all-out maximal lift is essential for weightlifting purposes. If by chance you say, "but, I've always been told 'you never hold your breath,'" I challenge you to do an all-out maximal lift while breathing. It's not possible. Your body is so tense and rigid on an all-out maximal lift that it can't breathe. If, by chance, you do a heavy lift and are able to breath, well, you didn't go heavy enough.

NON-MAXIMAL LIFTS

Following the sequences in this book, especially the Forever sequence, you are bound to come across breathing issues. Namely, you will find it hard to keep an adequate "breath" while completing the sequence. In that case, since these sequences—except the Partials sequence—use non-maximal weight, that is, light to medium weight, it shall be preferable to hyper-ventilate by taking a succession of shallow breaths. This will enable you to keep going. However, do not go crazy here, as you can easily overdo it and get lightheaded.

TAPER-OFF PROGRESSION

Back to the table, first select your week(s) or month(s), then calculate the projected maximums, then select your reps. Lastly, select your weight values. A realistic weekly step can be a 2.5-pound increment. However, if someone makes a lot of gains early on and then tapers off slowly, a better increment would be one that reflects this. An example that reflects this is a 10-pound increment at first, then a pound down a week.

WEEK	WEIGHT x REPS	PROJECTED MAX
1	295 x 1	295 (0)
2	229 x 10	305 (10)
3	247 x 8	314 (9)
4	272 x 5	322 (8)
5	293 x 3	329 (7)
6	276 x 6	335 (6)
7	303 x 3	340 (5)
8	291 x 5	344 (4)
9	273 x 8	347 (3)
10	262 x 10	349 (2)
11	350 x 1	350 (1)

MACRONUTRIENTS OF COMMON (PRISON) FOODS

FOOD TYPE	CALORIES	FIBER (G)	PROTEIN (G)	FAT (G)	CARBS (G)
1 LARGE TOMATO	33	2	2	0	7
1 CUP (145G) PEAS	117	7	8	1	21
1 CUP CORN	132	4	5	2	29
1 CUP CELERY	16	1.6	7	0.17	3
1 CUP GREEN BEANS	34	4	2	0	8
1 CUP POTATO	104	4	2	0	26
1 CUP RED POTATO	104	2	2	0	24
1 CUP JICAMA	46	6	1	0	11
1 CUP CARROT	52	4	1	0	12
1 CUP BEETS	58	4	2	0	13
1 CUP RADISH	19	2	1	0	4
1 CUP BROCOLLI	31	2	3	0	6
1 CUP CAULIFLOWER	25	3	2	0	5
1 CUP SPINACH	7	1	1	0	1
1 CUP LETTUCE	10	1	1	0	2
1 WHOLE CUCUMBER	45	2	2	0	11
1 CUP ONION	64	3	2	0	15
1OZ ALMONDS	167	3	6	15	5
1OZ CASHEWS	161	1	4	13	9
1OZ PEANUTS	164	2	7	14	6
1OZ SUNFLOWER	168	3	5	14	7
1 CUP BLACK BEANS	227	15	15	1	41
FOOD TYPE	CALORIES	FIBER (G)	PROTEIN (G)	FAT (G)	CARBS (G)

FOOD TYPE	CALORIES	FIBER (G)	PROTEIN (G)	FAT (G)	CARBS (G)
1OZ PINTO BEANS	97	4	6	0	18
1 CUP SPLIT PEA	231	16	16	1	41
1 CUP LENTILS	230	16	18	1	40
1 MED APPLE	95	4	0	0	25
1 MED BANANA	105	3	1	0	27
1 LARGE ORANGE	86	4	2	0	22
1 CUP WATERMELON	46	1	1	0	12
1 CAN TUNA	220	0	41	5	0
1 CUP WHITE RICE	242	0	4	0	53
1 CUP OATMEAL	160	4	6	4	32
1 CUP BELL PEPPER	30	3	1	0	7
1 CUP MILK 1%	102	0	8	2	13
½ CUP ICE CREAM	137	0	2	7	16
1OZ WHEY & CASEIN	109	0	22	1	3
1 SLICE WHEAT BREAD	69	2	4	2	12
1 WHOLE TORTILLA	70	2	3	0	20
1 CUP PASTA	221	3	8	1	43
4OZ TURKEY	128	0	28	1	0
1 EGG	71	0	6	5	0
4OZ CHICKEN	124	0	24	1	0
4OZ GROUND BEEF	240	0	20	16	0
1OZ BACON	128	0	3	13	0
1OZ ROAST BEEF	30	0	8	1	0
FOOD TYPE	CALORIES	FIBER (G)	PROTEIN (G)	FAT (G)	CARBS (G)

METABOLISM

In particular, resting metabolism is when you will burn most of your calories. By far one of the biggest and within your control influences on metabolism is muscle mass. Muscle mass will burn at least 35 calories a day per pound. In general, you can burn up to 50 to 100 calories a day per pound of muscle.

Body fat loss is threefold: First, putting on muscle mass raises the resting metabolism, therefore burning more calories. Second, calories are burned during the exercise. Third, the afterburn of exercise, when the body is burning calories recovering, repairing, and rebuilding the body.

There are three energy systems at work: The ATP-PC system (fast), the glycolytic system (medium), and the oxidative system (slow).

ATP-PC (fast) System: Can supply an intense burst of energy for about 10–12 seconds before it runs out; uses adenosine triphosphate (ATP).

Glycolytic System: Starts being put to use after about 10 seconds, when the ATP-PC system is depleted; primarily uses glucose from glycogen.

Oxidative System: Fat burning.

SOMATOTYPE

Endomorph: A person has a likeliness of being soft and squat.

Mesomorph: A person has a likeliness of being lean and muscular.

Ectomorph: A person has a likeliness of being very lean and thin.

Note: It is uncommon to find a pure archetypal somatotype. Commonly, people will be a mixture of these.

FAT DISTRIBUTION

For the average person, there are 25–30 billion fat cells. When it comes to the obese, there may be 50 billion or up to well over a 100 billion fat cells.

OVERTRAINED... NOW WHAT?

So, you didn't listen, and did many sets, plus took no time off, and are in an overtrained state. Now what? Well now first off, take a week or two off. Right now. *Do no exercise or similar activities*.

Second, de-load by doing the Forever sequence with 0–50% of your max. *The lower you start off with the better*. Keep at it for at least a workout cycle, up to a month or two.

TRUE STORY

Before committing myself to high-intensity training, I was a classic "over-trainer," and a bad one at that. My workout program then was no days off, I repeat no days off, for a whole 9 months. On top of that, it was a push, pull, legs routine where I came out to the weight pile three times a day.

When the rug was pulled from under my feet, boy was it pulled from under me. Injuries were constant, swelling was a daily struggle, plus my precious gains were taken away. Once that happened, I began to question myself, in particular whether I had some "rare" muscular disease.

I didn't. I was in an over-trained state, and a bad one at that. Then, I read high-intensity books that saved my life (weight-lifting wise). I was done overtraining and lifting heavy, and turned my back on it. Well, I did a 6-month de-load where I did the Forever sequence for only a third of my prior heavy weight on my main lifts, which was about 95 pounds. That's 95 pounds bench-press, 95 pounds full squat, and 95 pounds deadlift.

A buddy of mine to whom I'm forever thankful, got me back into lifting heavy. After such a long de-load with plenty of time off, I returned back to heavy weightlifting. My first time back to heavy bench-press was 255 pounds, full squat was 275 pounds, and deadlift was 355 pounds. These maxes were preserved from de-loading and lifting 95 pounds using the Forever sequence.

If I hadn't done so, there is no telling how much lower my maxes would have been due to the overtrained state I was in. Now, was six months off of heavy weight really required? Probably not. Without going back in time, there is no way of knowing. Point is, de-loading with 0–50% of your max using the Forever sequence works.

PART THREE

MYTHS

RESULTS

So many workouts and weightlifting programs are driven by anything except for what's most important; *results.*

So long as you are not in an overtrained state, you will see results immediately. Yes, immediately. Your indicator of success will be and should always be *results*.

People mistake many of these indicators as a sign of success. You'll commonly hear "oh, but I'm so sore" or "I haven't gone up in strength, but I could feel I've put on muscle" or "but, I feel I got such a good pump." Undoubtedly one of my biggest challenges will be to convince you to do less, not more. Part of that challenge will be in that you need to feel you got a good workout, or not at all. If you've plateaued or lost strength, tell me, how can you trust your feelings?

"But, I'm so sore"

I'm guilty of this one in the past. I was a sore chaser. In a nutshell, soreness is only an indicator of the inflammation response, not the building of muscle—although, that might occur anyway.

TRUE STORY

For a time, like many others, I was one who could bench-press more than he could squat. Until the November of 2018, when my squat finally surpassed my bench-press. Keep in mind that the previous month, I had done my maxes and was at 285 pounds for bench-press and at 265 pounds for the full squat.

Come the end of November, to my surprise, I was squatting 265 pounds for 3 repetitions. My surprise was due to the fact that for that whole month, my legs were not sore once, while my chest on the other hand was sore every time I had worked it out. I had lost sight of what truly matters to judging the success of my workouts up until that month, which is that *results should always be an indicator of success*.

"I haven't gone up in strength, but I could feel I put on muscle"

This is one of those 'you need one to get the other' situations. Yes, it's possible to put on some strength and not go up in muscle. However, you cannot go up in muscle but not strength. Most importantly, "how do you feel you put on muscle?"

"But I got such a good pump"

Being a "pump chaser" is just as bad as being a "sore chaser" φor much the same reasons. Having a pump is just an indicator of having blood rushing through your muscles, nothing else.

"But I'm losing so much weight"

Unless you're doing a competition, weight loss should be slow and steady. It's not safe to lose more than 2 pounds a week. In fact, the science behind rapid weight loss is that it can lower your resting metabolic rate to the point that it does more harm than good.

"But I didn't get a good sweat"

Being a sweat chaser is another way you'll be led to overtraining. Sweat is just an indicator of the body maintaining a healthy normal body temperature, nothing else.

MYTH: YOU HAVE TO WORK OUT FOR HOURS

I hear it all the time. "I was working out for 2–3 hours and looked great," "I had the best results" or "I was in the best shape of my life, while running a marathon a day."

First of all, yeah, you had it in you to run and workout all this time, what were you, unemployed and rich to maintain all that and never have anything else to do? The reason people always say "I used to" is because it was unsustainable (however much of what they said was really true), otherwise you'd still be doing it.

When someone tells me they do 2–3-hour workouts, I already know what they really did. They did 30–45 minutes of lifting with a total of 2 and more hours of rest in between sets. Hmm, let's see, how is that really 2–3 hours of "working out?" And as far as "marathon" style "cardio," I can walk 26.2 miles about as fast as some of these people "run" a marathon.

The bottom line is this: train intensely for the stimulation needed to get anabolic muscle building effects and do the aerobic amount needed to get the EPOC effect. That simple. It shouldn't take more than a few minutes a day, if that.

OVERCOMING THE FEAR OF THE WEIGHT PILE

DECEMBER 2017

It's the day-room of Alpha unit, a mental health pod at the Deer Ridge Correctional Institution. I'm pacing around as usual, trying to avoid the scale, since the last time I weighed myself was at Medical, and at that time, I had been informed I weighed 185 pounds.

Seeing as how I came into prison weighing 165 pounds, well, that had placed me at 20 pounds overweight, at least. My stomach and chest have taken the most damage, as I now wore a sweater everywhere. However, people still saw through it and some called me "Fat Bobby."

"Oh, what the hell, why not just walk right over and weigh myself?" I do just that and "oh my goodness!" I weighed 205 pounds. Back when I weighed 165 pounds, the USN Navy informed me that I had 15 or so percent of body fat. So, if my calculations were correct, that placed me at about 25 pounds of body fat. So, now, that was 25 pounds, plus the 40 pounds I've gained, which puts me at 65 pounds of pure fat.

3RD WEEK OF DECEMBER 2017

I finally work up the nerve to go out to the yard, which is just 20 feet from my cell, and workout. The yard has six power racks, a body-weight station, and some cable machines, and these are surrounded by a track that is 11 laps to a mile.

Okay, time to get serious. My first exercise is pull-ups. I walk to the body-weight station and pull my fat ass up for one pull-up. I attempt a second one—nada, couldn't budge my fat ass up a second time. I need the next five minutes to catch my breath, off of just that one pull-up.

Well, that's one exercise down. Next, is the bench-press. My good ole' friend, the bench-press. I used to press over 300 pounds back in the day. I walk over to the power rack with a 35-pound plate on each side for a total of 115 pounds, and pump out 7 repetitions. I'm already sore. The beating in my chest from that one set goes on for over five minutes.

Now, it's time for some squats. I walk over to the power rack with one wheel on each side for a total of 135 pounds. Easy enough, just get under the wheel and pump out some squats. I squat for no more than 5 repetitions and I get so out of breath I have to stop. This time, my heart pounds for over ten minutes. Honestly, I feared a heart attack the whole time. I stop, and the next time I work out again would be over 3 months later.

APRIL FOOL'S DAY 2018

It all started as an April Fool's dare. I had talked such a big talk to my cellmate about how much weight I used to lift and how much I used to run when I was 17, so on April first, he finally got tired of my bolstering. He said, "well, why don't you prove it then?" to which I replied, "I will and I'll start today." By the end of April, I would've increased my bench-press to 225 pounds, my squat to 225 pounds, and my pull-ups to 2.

DECEMBER 2018

Just under 9 months since I started working out. On the yard, there are carved-out walkways in the snow to the weight pile. It's the worst winter since I've been down. The snow is about chest level. Luckily, the rec orderlies have cleared the pile of the snow.

I walk up to the power rack that maxes out at 305 pounds. After a brief warm up, I'm at 305 pounds. Nobody's around, nobody to see me fail if I can't get this 305-pound beast off of me. If I get stuck, I'd have to shimmy the weight off side-to-side until all the plates fall off—a trick I'm not proud of learning.

Okay. I un-rack the 305. I take a deep breath and hold my breath, bringing the weight down to my chest. The easy parts over, now's the hard part to push it up. I push close to halfway up with no problem. At halfway there, I stall momentarily and think to myself, "it's all going to come crashing down on me now."

But I manage to clear the weight up and rack it. The lift was good.

EXERCISE JOURNAL AND NOTES

www.ingramcontent.com/pod-product-compliance
Ingram Content Group UK Ltd.
Pitfield, Milton Keynes, MK11 3LW, UK
UKHW061706190726
13853UKWH00008B/2431